Amazing ways to Live Long and Healthy
How to Live and Not Die

Catherine J. Puyear

Table of content

Chapter 1

The Ultimate Guide to Metabolic Health

Metabolic health can be improved by continuously making decisions that maintain glucose levels in a steady and healthy range. Metabolism is the collection of biological systems that create energy from our diet and environment to fuel every function in the human body. Metabolic health is a word to explain how effectively we create and process energy in the body.

Glucose is a fundamental precursor for energy in the body and has to be strictly managed for metabolism to perform correctly.

Metabolic health may be enhanced by constantly making decisions that maintain glucose levels in a steady and healthy range and reduce big glucose fluctuations.

These options may include picking meals that don't produce huge spikes in glucose, exercising regularly, obtaining quality sleep, controlling stress, adding in minerals and foods that help our digestion of glucose, and avoiding environmental contaminants that are known to disturb metabolic function.

Poor metabolic health is connected with poorer brain function, energy, memory, mood, skin health, fertility, and risk for chronic illness.
As a nation, our metabolic health is poor, with 88% of the American population demonstrating at least some metabolic abnormality.
Metabolic dysfunction underlies most chronic illnesses.

Metabolism is the collection of biological systems that create energy from our diet and environment to fuel every single cell in the body. When these energy-producing processes work smoothly, we have optimum metabolic health.

Since all cells in the body need energy to operate, metabolic health is essential for well-being.

Why would someone desire to enhance their metabolic health?

Stable and consistent energy throughout the day?

Sharp memory and recall

Sustained exercise endurance

Fat-burning abilities and healthy weight

Stable mood reduced anxiety and despair

Clear skin and fewer wrinkles

Improved fertility

Improved sexual health

A high-functioning immune system

Lower risk of chronic illnesses including diabetes, Alzheimer's disease, obesity, fatty liver disease, heart disease, stroke, and more

What is Metabolic Health?

Clinically speaking, metabolic health is characterized by ideal levels of five markers: blood sugar, triglycerides, high-density lipoprotein (HDL) cholesterol, blood pressure, and waist circumference—without requiring medication. We can improve most of these signs by continuously making decisions that maintain glucose levels in a steady and healthy range.

The opposing situation is known as metabolic syndrome when patients exhibit three or more of the following traits:

A waistline of 35 inches for ladies and 40 inches for males

Fasting glucose ≥ 100 mg/dL

HDL cholesterol less than 40 mg/dL

Triglycerides exceeding 150 mg/dL

High blood pressure (130/85 or greater)

Can You Improve Your Metabolic Health?
We frequently speak about metabolic fitness, since fitness is neither an innate attribute nor something that "happens to us." Rather, fitness is something that can increase when we put in constant labor and training. And much as with physical fitness, metabolic fitness improves when we put in the effort.

Let's use the example of beginning a running program to increase our physical fitness to run a marathon. Our first jog isn't going to be 26.2 miles; it's likely going to be a brief slog. But, when we lace up our shoes each day, hit the street, and measure our progress over time, we see and feel growth.

We notice minor modifications in our bodies: our breathing can grow easier when we run up hills, our muscles get more defined, and maybe our mood improves. We could measure our distance with Strava or our heart rate with a Fitbit and feel thrilled when these numbers start to improve. As the weeks of running continuously, it is apparent that our physical fitness is increasing.

On the other hand, if we decide to take a few months off from training, physical fitness would certainly decline: those hard-earned muscles may weaken, and we'd likely feel more winded the first time we go back out there.

The metabolism is no different. If we make everyday decisions that support metabolic processes, we will adjust to acquire improved metabolic fitness. We may not see our muscles expand, but within our bodies, the tiny machinery involved in turning fat and glucose into energy grows more efficient. While being physically fit needs constant exercise, becoming metabolically fit includes consistent wise choices about nutrition (including what to eat, when to eat, and how to pair meals), sleep, stress management, physical activity, and exposure to metabolism-disrupting environmental pollutants. Our current level of metabolic fitness is highly dynamic and largely in our control.

Just like we can track metrics of physical fitness to keep us informed, on track, and motivated, we can also now track our metabolic fitness. Since glucose is the primary energy-building block for our metabolism, tracking this biomarker can give us useful insight into our level of metabolic fitness.

And, just like with physical fitness, we can see meaningful improvements in our lives even if we haven't won an Olympic gold medal. Fitness is a spectrum and any tiny bit of progress is a gain. As with other functions in the body, there is no "on-off" button for metabolic health. We are neither "healthy" nor "unhealthy." Rather, we are on a metabolic continuum, and our choices—coupled with our genes—determine where we stand each day.

How Does Glucose Relate to Metabolic Health?

Glucose is a basic sugar that is a breakdown product of the carbs that we ingest. When glucose enters the circulation, it signals to the pancreas to produce insulin, a hormone that instructs cells to absorb glucose. Some of this glucose is metabolized by the mitochondria to generate energy (called ATP) that our cells may utilize. Excess glucose is stored in the muscle and liver as glycogen, and may also be converted to triglycerides and stored in fat cells.

When our systems require energy, we may tap into glucose from the circulation, store glycogen in the muscles or liver, or we can even generate fresh glucose from other molecules like amino acids (breakdown products of proteins) (breakdown products of proteins). Aside from utilizing glucose for creating energy, humans can also break down stored fat to produce energy, and convert protein breakdown products to energy.

However, when our bodies are taxed with processing too much dietary glucose over long periods, it throws off the balance of these processes and leads to health problems. First, chronic excess glucose causes the repeated release of insulin. High amounts of insulin may, over time, lead cells to become "numb" to insulin's impact, a phenomenon called insulin resistance.

When this happens, less glucose can get into the cells, so circulating glucose rises. Second, high insulin levels block stored fat from being broken down and used for energy. So, strangely, too much energy in the form of glucose causes us to have greater problems utilizing energy properly.

Aside from these concerns, excess glucose in the circulation causes inflammation (immune activation), oxidative stress (an overflow of harmful free radicals in the body), and glycation (glucose being "stuck" to substances in the body and causing malfunction).

Given how many harmful impacts excess glucose may have, it is not a surprise that the bulk of prevalent chronic illnesses is founded on poor glucose management, including Type 2 diabetes, obesity, heart disease, stroke, dementia, infertility, and more. This is a very contemporary phenomenon: humans used to die of infectious illnesses and famine. Now we die of metabolic illness.

Why would that be? In the beginning, we (on average) consume roughly 10x more sugar per day than we did 100 years ago. Many of us don't even notice it, since sugar is so widespread in our food culture, and it wears many masks (link: 56 names for sugar) (link: 56 names for sugar). Imagine a manufacturer receiving 10x more shipments of raw material and attempting to merely "make it work." It wouldn't. The factory would fall apart. The machinery would break. The employees would oppose defending themselves.

This is what is happening to our bodies. Additionally, too much dietary fat can impair glucose processing; in fact, excess saturated fat impairs the function of the insulin receptor, leading to more circulating glucose.

In summary, extra energy precursors like glucose and fat gum up our bodies' machinery, and are the source of a great amount of sickness and misery worldwide. "Our lives now are unrecognizable compared to earlier centuries."

Currently, just 12% of Americans have excellent metabolic health. The remaining 88% have one or more signs that suggest that individuals have metabolic dysfunction and that their bodies are not able to consume and metabolize fat and carbs adequately.

In this research study, to be called "metabolically healthy," you had to have normal blood glucose, triglycerides (a kind of fat that is created from excess glucose), high-density lipoprotein cholesterol, blood pressure, and waist circumference, without the need for drugs.

What is Glucose?
Glucose is a simple carbohydrate, a monosaccharide, which implies it is a single sugar. We receive glucose from the food we consume.

What are the Consequences of Poor Metabolic Health?

What do metabolic dysfunction and poor metabolic health and fitness look like? It may be both overt and subtle.

Overtly, metabolic dysfunction looks like obesity (dysfunctional body fat storage, often measured by BMI), insulin resistance and diabetes (dysfunctional glucose processing), non-alcoholic fatty liver disease (dysfunctional management of glucose and fat in the liver), cancer (cancer cells thrive on excess sugar), Alzheimer's disease (now being called type 3 diabetes, with evidence of insulin resistance in the brain), cardiovascular diseases like heart attack and stroke (damage to vessels from inflammation and excess glucose), and chronic kidney disease (vessels of the kidney impaired by excess glucose) (vessels of the kidney impaired by excess glucose).

But more subtly, poor metabolic health can look like the full spectrum of daily pain points of modern living that keep us from reaching our full potential and goals: fatigue, brain fog, depression, anxiety, lack of exercise endurance, infertility, balding, erectile dysfunction, acne, chronic pain, increased appetite, and more.

The point is this: because every cell type requires energy to operate, metabolic dysfunction doesn't discriminate. When our metabolic health is not ideal, the impacts may be extensive and varied, subtle and overt.

What are Risk Factors for Poor Metabolic Health?
Previously, we highlighted that current research suggests that 88% of Americans are not metabolically healthy. What's more, 71.6% of the US are overweight or obese, 120 million Americans are living with

diabetes and prediabetes, and 25-40% of the US suffers from mostly avoidable non-alcoholic fatty liver disease (NAFLD) (NAFLD).

Why are we witnessing such a high frequency of poor metabolic health and its downstream consequences? Our genetic makeup has not materially altered in the period that these illnesses have become prevalent, but our lives are unrecognizable as compared to past eras.

Some of the risk factors for our low metabolic fitness (all of which are controllable in our individual lives):
Chronic "overnutrition": We are exposed to a considerably larger quantity of food than ever previously in history, and our cellular factories haven't developed to deal with this level of incoming energy. We consume roughly 10x more sugar per day than we did 100 years ago.

This stimulates the pancreas repeatedly to create insulin (the hormone that helps cells take up glucose), and the cells gradually develop insensitive to this hormone. The liver becomes dysfunctional as excess glucose is converted to fat and stored in it, while the muscles become insulin resistant and unable to utilize glucose adequately. Even "normal weight" persons may have this type of dysfunction.

We are more sedentary than ever.
We tend to get less sleep, which has substantial ramifications for our capacity to metabolize energy.
Our environmental and synthetic toxin exposure damages mitochondria and metabolism.

The bulk of energy consumption among persons in the US comes from ultra-processed foods and drinks.
The experience of psychological stress appears to be increasing, which creates a

hormonal cascade that promotes storage, rather than use, of energy.

Eating late at night and eating often — normal activities in contemporary life — might result in greater levels of insulin that inhibit fat use for energy in the body.

Five metabolic-health myths—busted

We clarify some of the most frequent myths about metabolism and blood sugar to help you make better food and lifestyle choices.

How does Blood Sugar Reflect Metabolic Health?

If your metabolic machinery is operating effectively, your blood sugar reactions will look like this:

Minimal increase of glucose after meals

A rapid return of glucose to baseline after meals

Maintaining 24-hour glucose levels in a reasonably narrow and safe range

Keeping fasting glucose (glucose levels measured after ingesting no calories for at least 8 hours) in a healthy, low-risk range

What should your glucose levels be? Here's the complete guide to healthy blood sugar ranges
We explored the scholarly literature to offer more insights into what glucose levels could be best for healthy health.

Poor metabolic health appears more irregular, spiky, and high. Some of this could relate to our body's sensitivity to insulin, knowing that excessive exposure to carbohydrates and lipids might increase insulin resistance. When our cells become insulin resistant, they have greater difficulty taking in glucose, hence we may see:
Higher glucose peaks after meals
Longer intervals of high glucose after meals
Morning glucose levels higher than desired
"Basal" glucose (the glucose level in between meals) is high

More up-and-down glucose fluctuation throughout the day

Paying attention to how your blood sugar reacts to your food and lifestyle is a fantastic first step in enhancing metabolic health. A continuous glucose monitor is one of the greatest instruments for this task, but you may also accomplish it using a glucometer.

Given that there are numerous and contradicting health and nutritional signals coming at us from all sources, it might be good to have an objective data stream that informs us continually whether we are remaining on track in maintaining glucose steady.

By measuring glucose, we can see how diet and lifestyle decisions are directly influencing our metabolic health, with a tight feedback loop that supports quick learning and the capacity to modify. People might have quite diverse glycemic reactions to the same food, so understanding how you are individually impacted by a given meal is crucial.

There are several techniques for boosting metabolic health, ranging from eating less refined meals to matching carbs with protein, exercising, to participating in mindfulness practice. Behaviors like walking after meals, consuming fiber, and frequent exercise will certainly lead to improved grades. If you didn't sleep well or ate items that raise your blood sugar, you may find your metabolic fitness score lower, between 40 and 60. The typical Levels user has a metabolic fitness score between 70 and 80.

Three Key Metabolic Health Takeaways

Metabolic fitness takes practice.
Developing metabolic fitness and sustaining excellent metabolic health needs work and repetition. Just like the process of progress

in sports, martial arts, meditation, or any other activity, constancy is vital.
We can all improve.

Some of us are closer to our metabolic health objectives than others, but no one is fully metabolically healthy. The body is a dynamic mechanism and metabolic optimization is a daily, constant activity.

You are in charge.
Your metabolic fitness level is not a predefined attribute, it's a description of your present state: continually in flux and always customizable. You can make easy, educated choices each day that can enhance the measurements that characterize your metabolic health.

Chapter 2

Heart-healthy diet: 8 steps to prevent heart disease

Although you may know that eating certain foods might raise your heart disease risk, altering your dietary habits is typically tricky. Whether you have years of poor eating under your belt or you just wish to fine-tune your diet, here are eight heart-healthy diet guidelines. Once you know which foods to consume more of and which foods to restrict, you'll be on your way toward a heart-healthy diet.

1. Control your portion size
How much you eat is equally as essential as what you consume. Overloading your plate, having seconds, and eating until you feel filled might lead to consuming more calories than you should. Portions provided at restaurants are typically more than anybody needs.

Following a few basic guidelines to reduce food portion size will help you shape up your diet as well as your heart and waistline: Use a tiny dish or bowl to help regulate your servings.

Eat more low-calorie, nutrient-rich meals, like fruits and vegetables
Eat lesser quantities of high-calorie, high-sodium items, such as refined, processed, or fast foods.
It's also vital to keep track of the number of servings you consume. Some things to bear in mind:

A serving size is a set quantity of food, defined by conventional measures such as cups, ounces, or pieces. For example, one serving of spaghetti is around 1/3 to 1/2 cup, or about the size of a hockey puck. A serving of meat, fish, or chicken is around 2 to 3 ounces, or about the size and thickness of a deck of cards.

The suggested amount of servings of each food type may vary based on the particular diet or recommendations you're following. Judging serving size is a taught skill. You may need to use measuring cups and spoons or a scale until you're satisfied with your judgment.

2. Eat more veggies and fruits

Vegetables and fruits are rich providers of vitamins and minerals. Vegetables and fruits are also low in calories and high in nutritional fiber. Vegetables and fruits, like other plants or plant-based diets, contain chemicals that may help prevent cardiovascular disease. Eating more fruits and vegetables may help you cut less on higher-calorie meals, such as meat, cheese, and snack foods.

Featuring veggies and fruits in your diet might be straightforward. Keep veggies cleaned and chopped in your refrigerator for fast snacking. Keep fruit in a bowl in your kitchen so that you'll remember to eat it. Choose meals that contain vegetables or fruits as the major elements, such as vegetable stir-fry or fresh fruit blended into salads.

Fruits and vegetables to pick Fruits and vegetables to limit
Fresh or frozen veggies and fruits
Low-sodium canned veggies
Canned fruit packed with juice or water
Coconut
Vegetables in creamy sauces
Fried or breaded veggies
Canned fruit packed with thick syrup
Frozen fruit with sugar added

3. Select whole grains
Whole grains are rich sources of fiber and other nutrients that have a role in managing blood pressure and heart health. You may boost the number of whole grains in a heart-healthy diet by making easy

adjustments for refined grain products. Or be adventuresome and try a new whole grain, such as whole-grain farro, quinoa, or barley.

4. Limit unhealthy fats
Limiting how much saturated and trans fats you consume is a key step to decreasing your blood cholesterol and lowering your risk of coronary heart disease. A high blood cholesterol level may lead to a buildup of plaques in the arteries, termed atherosclerosis, which can raise the risk of heart attack and stroke.

The American Heart Association recommends this advice for how much fat to eat in a heart-healthy diet:
The type of fat recommended
Saturated fat
Less than 6% of total daily calories.* If you're consuming 2,000 calories a day, that's around 11 to 13 grams.

Transfat to Avoid

*Note: The 2020-2025 Dietary Guidelines for Americans propose reducing saturated fat to less than 10% of total daily calories.
There are easy strategies to cut down on saturated and trans fats:
Trim fat from meat or pick lean meats with less than 10% fat.
Use less butter, margarine, and shortening while cooking and serving.

Use low-fat substitutes wherever feasible for a heart-healthy diet. For example, top a baked potato with low-sodium salsa or low-fat yogurt rather than butter, or use the sliced whole fruit or low-sugar fruit spread over toast instead of margarine.

Check the food labels of cookies, cakes, frostings, crackers, and chips. Not only are these items lacking in nutritional value, several — even those labeled reduced fat —

may include trans fats. Trans fats are no longer authorized to be added to meals, however, older goods may still contain them. Trans fats may be indicated as partly hydrogenated oil on the ingredient label.

Fats to pick
Olive oil
Canola oil
Vegetable and nut oils
Margarine, trans-fat-free
Cholesterol-lowering margarine, such as Benecol, Promise Activ, or Smart Balance
Nuts, seeds
Avocados
Butter
Nondairy creamers
Hydrogenated margarine with shortening
Cocoa butter, found in chocolate
Coconut, palm, cottonseed, and palm kernel oils

When you do use fats, pick monounsaturated fats, such as olive oil or canola oil. Polyunsaturated fats, found in some seafood, avocados, nuts, and seeds, also are wonderful options for a heart-healthy diet. When utilized instead of saturated fat, monounsaturated and polyunsaturated fats may help decrease your total blood cholesterol. But moderation is key. All forms of fat are rich in calories.

a simple method to add healthy fat (and fiber) to your diet is to use ground flaxseed. Flaxseeds are little brown seeds that are abundant in fiber and omega-3 fatty acids. Studies have revealed that flaxseed decreases harmful cholesterol levels in certain individuals. You may crush the flaxseeds in a coffee grinder or food processor and add a teaspoon of them to yogurt, applesauce, or hot porridge.

5. Choose low-fat protein sources
Lean meat, poultry and fish, low-fat dairy products, and eggs are some of the greatest sources of protein. Choose lower-fat choices, such as skinless chicken breasts rather than

fried chicken patties and skim milk rather than whole milk.

Fish is a healthy alternative to high-fat meats. Certain forms of fish are rich in omega-3 fatty acids, which help decrease blood fats called triglycerides. You'll find the biggest quantities of omega-3 fatty acids in cold-water fish, such as salmon, mackerel, and herring. Other sources include flaxseed, walnuts, soybeans, and canola oil.

Legumes – beans, peas, and lentils — also are superb, low-fat sources of protein and contain no cholesterol, making them suitable alternatives for meat. Substituting plant protein for animal protein — for example, a soy or bean burger for a hamburger — can decrease fat and cholesterol consumption and increase fiber intake.

Proteins to pick Proteins to restrict or avoid\sLow-fat dairy products, such as skim or low-fat (1%) milk, yogurt, and cheese

Eggs
Fish, particularly fatty, cold-water fish, such as salmon
Skinless poultry
Legumes
Soybeans and soy products, such as soy burgers and tofu
Lean ground meats
Full-fat milk and other dairy products
Organ meats, such as liver
Fatty and marbled meats
Spareribs
Hot dogs and sausages
Bacon
Fried or breaded meats

6. Limit or minimize salt (sodium) (sodium)
Eating too much salt may contribute to high blood pressure, a risk factor for heart disease. Limiting salt (sodium) is an

essential aspect of a heart-healthy diet. The American Heart Association advises that:
Healthy individuals consume no more than 2,300 milligrams (mg) of sodium a day (approximately a teaspoon of salt) (about a teaspoon of salt)
Most individuals should consume no more than 1,500 mg of salt a day

Although lowering the amount of salt you add to meals at the table or while cooking is a smart beginning step, most of the salt you consume comes from canned or processed foods, such as soups, baked goods, and frozen dinners. Eating fresh ingredients and cooking homemade soups and stews might lower the amount of salt you ingest.

If you appreciate the convenience of canned soups and prepared meals, seek ones with no added salt or reduced sodium. Be skeptical of items that claim to be reduced in sodium because they are seasoned with sea salt instead of conventional table salt -

sea salt has the same nutritional value as regular salt.

Another strategy to decrease the amount of salt you consume is to pick your condiments wisely. Many condiments are available in reduced-sodium variants. Salt replacements may give a taste to your dish with less sodium.

Low-salt foods to pick

Herbs and spices

Salt-free seasoning mixes

Canned soups or prepared meals with no added salt or reduced sodium

Reduced-salt variants of condiments, such as reduced-salt soy sauce and reduced-salt ketchup

High salt goods

Table salt

Canned soups and prepared dishes, such as frozen dinners

Tomato juice

Condiments such as ketchup, mayonnaise, and soy sauce
Restaurant meals

7. Plan ahead: Create daily menus

Create daily meals using the six ideas outlined above. When picking meals for each meal and snack, prioritize vegetables, fruits, and whole grains. Choose lean protein sources and healthy fats, and minimize salty meals. Watch your portion sizes and provide diversity to your food options.

For example, if you eat grilled salmon one evening, try a black bean burger the following night. These aids guarantee that you'll acquire all of the nutrients the body requires. Variety also makes meals and snacks more intriguing.

8. Allow yourself an occasional treat

Allow yourself an indulgence now and again. A candy bar or handful of potato chips won't disrupt your heart-healthy diet. But don't let that turn into an excuse for giving up on your healthy-eating strategy. If overindulgence is the exception, rather than the norm, you'll balance things out over the long run. What's crucial is that you consume nutritious things most of the time.

Include these eight principles into your life, and you'll discover that heart-healthy eating is both feasible and pleasurable. With forethought and a few easy modifications, you can eat with your heart in mind.

Chapter 3

Importance of sleep and exercise

9 Reasons to Get More Sleep
Getting a good night's sleep is vitally crucial for your health. It's just as vital as eating a balanced, healthy diet and exercising.
Though sleep demands vary from person to person, most individuals need between 7 and 9 hours of sleep every night. Yet, up to 35% of individuals in the United States don't get enough sleep.

Sleep deprivation may put your health and safety in danger, which is why you must prioritize and safeguard your sleep every day.

1. May help you maintain or decrease weight
Numerous studies have related short sleep — defined as sleeping less than 7 hours each night — with an increased risk of weight

gain and a higher body mass index (BMI) (BMI).

A 2020 investigation indicated that persons who slept less than 7 hours every night had a staggering 41% greater chance of becoming fat. Meanwhile, sleeping longer didn't enhance the danger.

The influence of sleep on weight growth is considered to be regulated by various variables, including hormones and the desire to exercise.
For instance, sleep loss raises levels of ghrelin and reduces levels of leptin. Ghrelin is a hormone that makes us feel hungry whereas leptin makes us feel full. This may lead us to feel hungry and overeat.

This is confirmed by several research that has demonstrated that sleep-deprived persons have a higher appetite and prefer to consume more calories.

What's more, to compensate for lack of energy, sleep deprivation may make you seek meals that are higher in sugar and fat, owing to their greater calorie content.

To make things worse, feeling fatigued after a night of too little sleep may leave you feeling uninspired to go to the gym, go for a stroll, or do any other physical activity you prefer. So, prioritizing sleep may maintain healthy body weight.

Short sleep duration is related to an increased risk of acquiring obesity and weight gain. Sleep deprivation may boost your hunger and drive you to consume more calories. For instance, you're more inclined to consume items heavy in sugar and fat.

2. Can enhance focus and productivity
Sleep is vital for numerous areas of brain function. Cognition, focus, productivity, and performance are all adversely impacted by sleep deprivation.

Particular research on overworked doctors gives an excellent illustration. It discovered that clinicians with moderate, high, and very high sleep-related impairment were 54%, 96%, and 97% more likely to report clinically significant medical mistakes.

On a related note, obtaining adequate sleep may enhance academic performance in children, adolescents, and young adults.
Finally, adequate sleep has been demonstrated to increase problem-solving abilities and boost memory performance in both children and adults
Good sleep may boost problem-solving abilities and improve memory. In contrast, insufficient sleep has been found to decrease cognitive function and decision-making ability.

3. Can enhance athletic performance
Sleep has been found to increase athletic performance.

Numerous studies have demonstrated that proper sleep may boost fine motor abilities, response speed, muscular power, muscular endurance, and problem-solving skills.

What's more, lack of sleep may raise your risk of injury and diminish your enthusiasm to exercise. So, getting adequate sleep may be exactly the thing you need to take your performance to the next level. Getting adequate sleep has been demonstrated to enhance several elements of sports and physical performance.

4. May strengthen your heart
Low sleep quality and duration may raise your chance of getting heart disease.
One review of 19 research indicated that sleeping less than 7 hours per day resulted in a 13% higher risk of dying from heart disease.

Another investigation indicated that compared with 7 hours of sleep, each 1-hour reduction in sleep was related to a 6% greater risk of all-cause death and heart disease.

What's more, brief sleep seems to raise the risk of high blood pressure, particularly in people with obstructive sleep apnea – a disorder characterized by disrupted breathing during sleep.

One research indicated that persons who slept less than 5 hours each night had a 61% greater chance of having high blood pressure than those who slept 7 hours. Interestingly, excessive sleep in adults — more than 9 hours — was also proven to raise the risk of heart disease and high blood pressure.

Sleeping less than seven hours every night is connected to an increased risk of heart disease and high blood pressure.

5. Affects sugar metabolism and type 2 diabetes risk

Short sleep is related to an increased risk of getting type 2 diabetes and insulin resistance — which is when your body cannot utilize the hormone insulin effectively.

A review of 36 trials with over 1 million participants indicated that extremely short sleep of fewer than 5 hours and short sleep of fewer than 6 hours increased the chance of acquiring type 2 diabetes by 48% and 18%, respectively.

It's considered that sleep deprivation may produce physiological changes like impaired insulin sensitivity, higher inflammation, and hunger hormone alterations, as well as behavioral changes like poor decision-making and more food consumption – all of which raise diabetes risk.

Plus, sleep deprivation is related to an increased risk of acquiring obesity, heart disease, and metabolic syndrome. These variables also raise your risk of diabetes. Many studies demonstrate a substantial relationship between chronic sleep deprivation and the risk of acquiring type 2 diabetes.

6. Poor sleep is connected to depression
Mental health difficulties, such as depression, are significantly connected to poor sleep quality and sleeping disorders. One research with 2,672 participants indicated that individuals with anxiety and depression were more likely to have worse sleep ratings than those without anxiety and depression.

In other research, those with sleeping problems including insomnia or obstructive sleep apnea also report greater rates of depression than those without.

If you have difficulties with sleep and feel your mental health has deteriorated, it's crucial to discuss this with your healthcare expert. Poor sleeping habits are closely connected to depression, especially for people with a sleeping condition.

7. Supports a healthy immune system
Lack of sleep has been found to damage immunological function. In one research, people who slept less than 5 hours each night were 4.5 times more likely to acquire a cold compared to those who slept more than 7 hours. Those who slept 5–6 hours were 4.24 times more likely.

Some research also shows that sufficient sleep may increase your body's antibody responses to influenza vaccinations.
Recently, early research suggests that obtaining adequate sleep before and after having a COVID-19 immunization may boost vaccine effectiveness. Still, further study is required to properly grasp this

probable relationship. Getting at least 7 hours of sleep will strengthen your immune function and help combat the common cold. It may also boost COVID-19 vaccination effectiveness, however additional study is required.

8. Poor sleep is related to higher inflammation
Poor sleep may have a substantial influence on inflammation in the body.
Sleep has a critical part in the regulation of our central nervous system. In particular, it's engaged in the stress-response systems known as the sympathetic nervous system and the hypothalamic-pituitary-adrenal (HPA) axis.

Sleep deprivation, particularly from disrupted sleep, is known to activate inflammatory signaling pathways and lead to greater levels of undesired indicators of inflammation, such as interleukin-6, and C-reactive protein.

Over time, chronic inflammation may trigger the development of numerous chronic illnesses, including obesity, heart disease, some forms of cancer, Alzheimer's disease, depression, and type 2 diabetes

Sleep disruption is associated with greater levels of inflammation. Over time, this may raise your chance of acquiring chronic diseases including heart disease, depression, and Alzheimer's disease.

9. Affects emotions and social relationships
Sleep deprivation decreases your capacity to control emotions and engage socially.
When we're exhausted, we have harder difficulty managing emotional outbursts and our behavior in front of others. Tiredness may also hinder our capacity to react to humor and convey empathy.

Plus, chronically sleep-deprived persons are more prone to withdraw from social gatherings and suffer loneliness. Prioritizing sleep may be a vital method to strengthen your connections with others and help you become more sociable.

If you battle with loneliness or emotional outbursts, don't be hesitant to seek out a friend, family member, or healthcare professional to obtain assistance. To discover more, browse this list of resources.

Sleep deprivation may affect your social skills and capacity to absorb emotions.

Lack of sleep may be hazardous

Not getting enough sleep may be detrimental to yourself and others.

When we're weary, our ability to concentrate on tasks, reflexes, and response speeds drop. Being excessively sleep-deprived is equivalent to having drunk excess alcohol.

Concerningly, the Centers for Disease Control and Prevention (CDC) states that 1 in 25 persons have fallen asleep at the wheel while driving. Those who slept less than 6 hours were most likely to fall asleep while driving. One 2018 research indicated that those who slept 6, 5, 4, or less than 4 hours had a chance of having an automobile collision that was 1.3, 1.9, 2.9, and 15.1 times greater, respectively.

This research reveals that your chance of an automobile accident climbs considerably with each hour of missing sleep.
Further, the CDC claims that being up for more than 18 hours is similar to having a blood alcohol level (BAC) of 0.05%. After 24 hours, this grows to 1.00%, which is beyond the legal driving limit.

In addition to increasing dangers linked with driving, lack of sleep may also raise the chance of occupational injury and mistakes. All in all, obtaining appropriate sleep is vital for everyone's safety.
Severe sleep deprivation raises your chances of being in a vehicle accident or being harmed at work. It may substantially

influence your capacity to make vital judgments.

The bottom line
Along with diet and exercise, taking care of your sleep is one of the cornerstones of health.
Lack of sleep is related to several detrimental health impacts, including an increased risk of heart disease, depression, weight gain, inflammation, and illness.
Though individual requirements vary, most research recommends that you should receive between 7 and 9 hours of sleep every night for the best health.
Just as you prioritize your food and physical activity, it's time to give sleep the attention it deserves.

7 major importance of exercise

Want to feel better, have more energy, and perhaps add years to your life? Just workout.

The health advantages of regular exercise and physical activity are hard to deny. Everyone benefits from exercise, regardless of age, sex, or physical ability.

Need more convincing to start moving? Check out these seven ways that exercise may lead to a happier, healthier you.

1. Exercise regulates weight

Exercise may help avoid excess weight gain or assist maintain weight reduction. When you participate in physical exercise, you burn calories. The more intensive the exercise, the more calories you burn.

Regular excursions to the gym are nice but don't panic if you can't find a significant block of time to work out every day. Any quantity of exercise is better than none at all. To gain the advantages of exercise, simply become more active throughout your day – take the stairs instead of the elevator or speed up your home tasks. Consistency is crucial.

2. Exercise combats health issues and disorders

Worried about heart disease? Hoping to avoid high blood pressure? No matter what your present weight is, being active improves high-density lipoprotein (HDL) cholesterol, the "good" cholesterol, and it reduces harmful triglycerides. This one-two punch maintains your blood flowing smoothly, which minimizes your risk of cardiovascular problems.

Regular exercise helps prevent or manage various health conditions and concerns, including:
Stroke
Metabolic syndrome
High blood pressure
Type 2 diabetes
Depression
Anxiety
Many forms of cancer
Arthritis Falls

It may also assist enhance cognitive function and helps lessen the risk of dying from all causes.

3. Exercise boosts mood
Need an emotional lift? Or need to destress after a hard day? A gym workout or brisk stroll might assist. Physical exercise activates several brain chemicals that may leave you feeling happier, calmer, and less stressed.

You may also feel better about your looks and yourself when you exercise consistently, which may raise your confidence and enhance your self-esteem.

4. Exercise promotes energy
Winded by supermarket shopping or domestic chores? Regular physical exercise may enhance your muscular strength and strengthen your endurance.
Exercise gives oxygen and nourishment to your tissues and helps your cardiovascular

system perform more effectively. And as your heart and lung health improve, you have more energy to undertake everyday duties.

5. Exercise promotes better sleep
Struggling to snooze? Regular physical exercise might help you fall asleep quicker, enjoy better sleep, and deepen your sleep. Just don't exercise too close to night, or you may be too stimulated to go to sleep.

6. Exercise brings the spark back into your sex life
Do you feel too exhausted or too out of shape to enjoy physical intimacy? Regular physical exercise may enhance energy levels and strengthen your confidence in your physical attractiveness, which may boost your sex life.

But there's much more to it than that. Regular physical exercise may boost arousal for women. And guys who exercise consistently are less likely to develop difficulties with erectile dysfunction than those who don't exercise.

7. Exercise can be enjoyable ... and sociable!
Exercise and physical exercise may be joyful. They provide you a chance to relax, enjoy the outdoors, or just indulge in things that make you happy. Physical exercise may also help you interact with family or friends in an enjoyable social situation.
So take a dancing class, go hiking trails, or join a soccer team. Find a physical activity you like, and simply do it. Bored? Try something new, or do something with friends or family.

The bottom line on exercise
Exercise and physical exercise are fantastic methods to feel better, increase your health, and have fun. For most healthy people, the U.S. Department of Health and Human Services recommends following exercise guidelines:

Aerobic activity. Get at least 150 minutes of moderate aerobic exercise or 75 minutes of intense aerobic activity a week, or a mix of moderate and strenuous activity.

The rules recommended that you carry out this activity over a week. To give even greater health advantages and to aid with weight reduction or sustaining weight loss, at least 300 minutes a week is advised. But even tiny quantities of physical exercise are useful.

Being active for little durations throughout the day might build up to bring health advantages.

Strength training. Do strength training exercises for all main muscle groups at least two times a week. Aim to execute a single set of each exercise with a weight or resistance level hard enough to exhaust your muscles after around 12 to 15 repetitions.

Moderate aerobic exercise includes activities such as brisk walking, bicycling, swimming, and mowing the yard. Vigorous aerobic exercise includes activities such as jogging, hard yard labor, and aerobic dance. Strength training may involve the use of weight machines, your weight, heavy bags, resistance tubing or resistance paddles in the water, or sports such as rock climbing.

If you want to reduce weight, reach particular fitness objectives or gain even more advantages, you may need to ramp up your moderate aerobic exercise even further. Remember to check with your doctor before beginning a new exercise program, particularly if you have any worries about your fitness, haven't exercised for a long time, or have chronic health conditions, such as heart disease, diabetes, or arthritis.

Chapter 4

13 Home remedy to increase life expectancy

Pharmacies are filled with medicines that promise to treat aging issues, yet some of the finest therapies are as natural as can be.

1. Water
Considering our body is made up of about 60 percent material, it seems plain sense that drinking adequate water should extend our life expectancy. "Drinking appropriate water to remain hydrated aids assist in digestion by keeping our stomach wet and lubricated, enabling our systems transfer nourishment to our cells, as well as in the eliminating of waste products,", it helps maintain our skin looking like a fresh grape vs a dry raisin."

Learn more about the advantages of drinking water. Some varieties of mineral water even provide magnesium, calcium, and phosphate.

2. Probiotics

"Probiotics are 'good' gut bacteria that provide many health benefits when part of a healthy diet and supplementation regimen, from immune system integrity to even producing certain vitamins,

"Research has also indicated that probiotics may help improve certain skin conditions like eczema, improve urinary tract health, and even lessen allergy symptoms,". While you can receive probiotics in many of the foods you consume, such as yogurt, kimchi, sauerkraut, and kefir, you may also enhance your daily intake with over-the-counter tablets.

3. Collagen peptides

You've certainly seen that collagen is a component in several beauty care products on the market today, but it's also present in the body naturally—in joints, bones, muscles, and tendons. "

It's the principal protein in the body that links tissues together and is also known as the body's scaffolding or supporting framework. The only difficulty is that, as we age, our body's synthesis of collagen begins to drop, which leads to outward indicators of aging such as wrinkles. Taking a collagen supplement, or ingesting any protein source high in proline and glycine, may assist improve your body's synthesis.

4. Turmeric
This golden ancient spice that gives curry its yellow color has a slew of anti-aging benefits, specifically anti-inflammatory and antioxidant protective perks. "The active ingredient, a compound called curcumin, has been found to prevent cognitive decline,

In other words, if you want to have a sharp mind through the decades, take turmeric. Studies also reveal turmeric helps treat many of the chronic ailments connected with aging including heart disease, Alzheimer's, diabetes, and cancer.

5. Vitamin D

If you're excellent about keeping out of the sun, the drawback might imply that you're not producing enough vitamin D—which is a hormone that plays a crucial part in practically all organ systems in the body. from prevention and treatment of heart disease, osteoporosis, muscular pain and weakness, joint pain, cognitive disorders, prevention of cold and flu, as well as the prevention of cancer and more, ideal levels of vitamin D in the blood should be approximately 120 nmol/L. "Older people also manufacture vitamin D less effectively than younger folks, hence supplementation is key."

6. Coconut oil

Coconut oil's advantages have been garnering a lot of attention—it is highly nutrient-dense, and people over the world utilize it as a natural cure for a multitude of maladies. coconut oil is a strong source of antioxidants, which help fight illnesses including cancer, heart disease, joint pain and inflammation, and aging. While it's not advisable to consume coconut oil in excessive quantities, owing to the possible negative feature that it may elevate bad LDL cholesterol, he urges customers to use it moderately in cooking to impart diverse tastes and provide diversity to their meals.

7. Omega-3 fatty acids

This heart-healthy fat is crucial to excellent health with a laundry list of advantages, such as enhancing eye, brain, and heart health and battling sadness and anxiety. "
Omega-3s found naturally in the diet in fatty fish like salmon, albacore tuna, mackerel, and sardines, and also in other sources like

chia, flax, and walnuts, are crucial for helping our body decrease inflammation, enhance heart health, and maintain good skin. "

Omega-3s are also crucial for brain functioning and some evidence suggests supplementation may be advantageous during pregnancy for fetal brain and eye development." customers are encouraged to take 2.5-3 grams of omega-3 per day, but to be careful to eat with meals to enhance absorption and reduce any gastrointestinal discomfort.

8. Green tea

For generations, healers have lauded this beverage as a lifespan promoter. One research published in the Annals of Epidemiology indicated that persons who drink green tea frequently are at a decreased risk for heart disease and premature mortality. Additionally, green tea has brain-boosting benefits—it helps to sharpen memory and increase concentration. Aim to consume one to two cups of green tea every day, preferably instead of your coffee.

9. Dark chocolate
Perhaps the mo, st tempting natural anti-aging cure, dark chocolate may keep you youthful owing to its strong antioxidant content. One research from the British Journal of Clinical Pharmacology found antioxidants in dark chocolate—mainly flavonoids—protect the brain against age-related cognitive loss. consuming dark chocolate consistently may have favorable benefits on the face by minimizing facial wrinkles, helping prevent sun exposure, and enhancing skin suppleness.

10. Blueberries\sThese luscious, spherical berries are more than delicious: They also contain an age-defying antioxidant called anthocyanin, which research has proven to possess potent anti-inflammatory benefits. "

In addition, blueberries stimulate brain communication, which promotes memory and aids regular levels, which may prevent neurodegeneration connected to Alzheimer's disease. "

Also, a study from the Harvard School of Public Health suggests frequent eating of blueberries may cut the risk of a heart attack in women by 32 percent."

11. CBD oil

You may have heard about the anxiety-reducing and sleep-enhancing advantages of CBD oil, but did you know it may enhance circulation, minimize heart troubles, and prevent the sort of high blood pressure connected to aging? "CBD oil made from cannabis has been demonstrated to lower blood pressure and improve circulation, however, there has not been a lot of research since cannabis has been outlawed for many years, "CBD oil eliminates the THC, which is the chemical that creates the 'high' for cannabis,"

12. Grapeseed oil
This oil, a byproduct of wine-making, also functions as an anti-aging cure. "
Used topically, grapeseed oil will strengthen hair strands when added to your usual hair conditioning routine and it can also be used as an all-natural makeup remover, which can also help minimize the appearance of small wrinkles owing to its great antioxidant capabilities. "

Grapeseed oil is high in vitamin E, vitamin and antioxidant recognized to be effective for the prevention of heart disease, especially when it's ingested as food." it is advisable to use a t straight or add a few drops to your favorite moisturizer or add a teaspoon to a skin mask of ripe avocados. These are the safest cooking oils to use for every sort of cuisine.

13. Yucca root

This root vegetable that's native to subtropical climes, especially South America, is rich in carbs and acts as a good source of fiber, vitamin C, potassium, and folate (a vital mineral for pregnant women) (an essential nutrient for pregnant women).

It also occurs to aid with creaky joints, an indication of arthritis. "Arthritis, like many illnesses, is inflammation-related, and yucca root extract happens to be an old natural therapy for inflammation. "Yucca is a good source of saponins, which may have anti-arthritic qualities by reducing intestinal protozoa which may play a role in joint inflammation."